The
"MADNESS"
of Usher's

**Coping with Vision and Hearing Loss
(Usher syndrome Type II)**

By Dorothy H. Stiefel

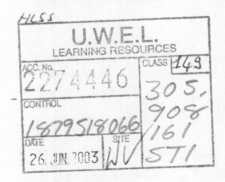
THE BUSINESS OF LIVING PUBLICATIONS

i

Library of Congress Catalog Card Number 90-90429

ISBN 1-879518-06-6

For further information, write to Dorothy H. Stiefel,
The Business of Living Publications, P. O. Box 8388,
Corpus Christi, Texas 78468-0388.

Printed in the United States of America

To my Mother,
I pay a posthumous tribute
for raising me with forthrightness
and discipline;
for teaching me to act
with honesty and integrity,
and to stand tall and erect
so I could face the world proudly.

ACKNOWLEDGMENTS

Many individuals have helped to make this book both a timely and enjoyable endeavor. I wish to thank Jim Young, of the National Writers' Club, for his personal encouragement and guidance in the field of self-publishing.

Special thanks go to my husband, Don, for his moral support and enduring patience, and to Edwin Jimenez who diligently kept my computer system operative and office supplies in readiness. Sincere appreciation is extended to my loyal friend, Linda Lindell, for reviewing the manuscript, and to Randall T. Jose, O.D., for assistance with the title page.

I am particularly grateful to Robert Gorman for "walking" with me, step by step, throughout the entire manuscript. Chapter by chapter, page by page, and down to sheer essence and momentum, he proved to be an invaluable critic. He knew very little about my dual disability and nothing of my "madness." As editing sessions continued, his sensitivity and interest grew, and his understanding increased. This cover-to-cover "trial run" was a unique experience, and enabled me to feel confident that I had accomplished my purpose in the production of this book.

TABLE OF CONTENTS

FOREWORD

The occurrence of retinitis pigmentosa and hearing impairment in the same individual was recognized as early as the late 1850s. However, the regular association of these two sensory impairments was not characterized until C. H. Usher, a Scottish ophthalmologist, described some forty families in a survey of hearing impairment and blindness in the United Kingdom in 1914. Usher clearly recognized the familial nature of these disorders and described two separate types, one in which children are born so severely deaf that they never develop speech and thus are "mute" and then develop retinitis pigmentosa in the latter half of the first decade of life. He also identified families in which a mild or moderate degree of hearing impairment was associated with retinitis pigmentosa of a later onset. This latter group has been called Usher syndrome Type II.

Although most individuals with retinitis pigmentosa have impairments only in their visual system, the additive association of hearing loss provides the most common recognized specific association with retinitis pigmentosa. It is estimated that the Usher syndromes comprise between six and ten percent of all individuals with retinitis pigmentosa. The estimated prevalence of these diseases in the population of the United States ranges from approximately 3.6 to 4.4 individuals per 100,000, although estimates as low as 5.6 individuals per million have been offered. About five or six percent of all deaf people of the United States have Usher syndrome of one type or the other.

Despite the long history of recognition of these diseases, many physicians, ophthalmologists, otorhinolargyngologists, and audiologists, are even yet unfamiliar with them. After reading this book, I cannot help but recall the many emotions of individuals and families whom I evaluate and counsel about these diseases. As with the diagnosis of any chronic, lifelong, and untreatable illness the discovery of the disease and the exploration of its complications leads to denial and occasionally rage. If the diagnosis has not been ascertained adequately, or if only one component of these sensory impairments is recognized, frustration and fear may follow the identification of the second component and the thoughts of possible abandonment of the individual to two handicaps. Parents of young children may express either shame or guilt that some august power has punished them for perceived sins. With appropriate counseling and proper, timely, and complete information from physicians, geneticists, and related support services, depression may then yield to compensation and contemplative reason.

As you read this book, be aware of your own experiences, whether you manage patients with Usher syndrome or whether you have or are relative to someone with one of these disorders. Physicians should advise affected individuals and their families to seek out complete and reliable knowledge and research that is being conducted and should refer them to regional and national resources for additional current information.

In the spring, 1990, two groups of investigators reported the assignment of the gene for Usher syndrome Type II to the long arm of chromosome 1. There is much work yet to be done to identify the specific nature of the gene and to determine whether this is a single disorder or the coincidental inheritance of two adjacent genes, one affecting visual function and one affecting hearing. As ophthalmologists, researchers, individuals, and families become aware that they are working on or part of real human problems and are sensitive to the spectrum of these diseases and the adaptive behaviors and life experiences of affected individuals, everyone will benefit. Today, unlike at any time in our past, there is now real hope for intervention. We now have the scientific skills to locate and isolate these genes and to understand their functions. More important, physicians and families have greater opportunities than ever to form partnerships to study together the progress of these disorders to benefit everyone. I commend to you the voice and the spirit of one courageous individual who incidentally also has Usher syndrome.

Richard A. Lewis, M. D.
Professor
Departments of Ophthalmology,
    Medicine, Pediatrics, and
    the Institute for Molecular
    Genetics
Baylor College of Medicine
Houston, Texas

x

INTRODUCTION

In both of my previous works I purposely omitted that I had a hearing loss in conjunction with retinitis pigmentosa (RP). I did not wish to give a false impression or to unwittingly imply that deafness always accompanies RP. I realized that readers might become fearful that they, also, would lose their hearing if I divulged that I had a dual disability. At this writing I still assure people that just because they have RP it does not mean they are also going to "go deaf."

This book has a direct, two-fold purpose: First, to alert, early in life, those persons who have hearing loss combined with RP and who may have Usher syndrome Type II; and second, to try to explain the "madness" to all who desire to be informed. I draw intimate attention to a pervading kind of anguish and confusion that disrupts normal behavior.

Throughout my human services work with the Texas Association of Retinitis Pigmentosa (TARP), correspondents continue to share their intense reactions to impending blindness: "overwhelming," "traumatic," "shocking," and "unbelievable." When deafness or hearing loss is a primary disability, the ominous news of "going blind" is perceived as catastrophic.

In many ways I think that having a dual disability is like being caught in a "twilight zone." Many people affected with Usher syndrome Type II walk a functional tightrope of deafness and blindness. Services for the deaf are not appropriate for a mild or moderate hearing impairment;

services for the blind and visually impaired often are not acceptable to those with decreasing, but still functional, vision.

In addition, families have immense struggles of their own. Fraught with guilt, well-meaning intentions often backfire. Spouses need a special "survival kit."

When you have a hearing problem all of your life, no one seems to attach severity to its ownership. I did not "grieve" my loss of hearing. It was "endowed." It came with skinny bowlegs, blond hair and a mother who constantly yelled at me.

Where does one look for guidance, for consolation, for peace of mind, and for stability? Available literature addresses the clinical aspects of a dual disability, but experiential anecdotes are superfluous, touching only the surface and not the "craziness."

Now, forty years after a diagnosis of RP in 1957 I, too, need reassurance. I have two minimally functioning major senses that threaten personal control over my life, my credibility as a functional person in mainstream society, and my sanity.

I have put myself on the "front lines" in ardent hope that my shared experiences of RP and hearing loss will be useful to those who are affected as well as those persons who are responsible for their welfare. Usher syndrome is an imbued battleground that requires a never-ending fight for daily survival. To my friends-in-kind I hope this book will serve as a realistic guide for personal survival.

1.

THE EARLY YEARS
Reflections

I have vivid childhood memories of long, hot and humid, summertime evenings, sitting on the front porch at night, on grandmother's lap watching fireflies in a jar, and the companionship of nearby commuter trains. Many evenings were so still there seemed not to be a whisper of a breeze nor a sound to catch my attention. But when the trains entered the railroad yard the "music" of their presence put me to sleep. My world was serene, and I was fascinated with what went on in the railroad yard at night.

I was very young when we lived for a time in an area parallel to the New Haven Railroad Line. Behind our one-story rental house was an enormous cyclone fence through which one could look far below and watch the commuter trains on their scheduled runs from New Rochelle north of us to New York City south of us. I distinctly remember the special sounds of the rumble of evening passenger trains from the City as they noisily hissed into low gear to approach the nearby station. The trains and their pattern of sounds made my small world alive and colorful. I also remember listening to the nightly freight cars switching tracks. A dairy farm close by loaded and moved its bottled milk by freight, so the sounds of several cars bumping and creaking back and forth clearly could be heard. It was as if the cars were trying to get comfortable. Then suddenly all would be quiet. I must have sensed it was also time for me to go to sleep.

2

Some evenings were so stifling that sleep was impossible. One memory is particularly clear. It was related to me many years ago by my grandmother. One unusually sultry evening I was put to bed earlier than usual. The heat was oppressive and no breeze came through the open window; nor was it time for the familiar chug-chug, clackety-clack and intermittent whines and whistles of the late evening shuttle trains. I must have felt alone. Also, I was not able to hear any household sounds, and the quietness must have given me a frightening sense of insecurity. I screamed for my mother.

Instantly, I felt cool hands soothing me as Mother lifted me out of the crib and carried me out of the house onto the front porch where the coolness of a faint breeze and Grandma's swaying rocker awaited me. It was a joyous escape from the fear I felt without the fullness and intricacies of lifesounds. Fireflies flitted about as I settled into my grandmother's lap.

"Look, Dorothy, see the 'lightning bugs?'" Grandma nudged me to see where she was pointing. (Of course I didn't know she did this when I was three, but evenings on the front porch were a special treat for many years.) Grandma always exclaimed playfully in succession, "See them, see them, see the 'lightning bugs!'" I think she must have enjoyed them as much as they thrilled me. I considered fireflies as magical. I would ask when I was a little older, "Where do the bugs get their lights?" They fascinated me until at age sixteen I could no longer find them. Little did I know that night blindness had snuffed out their profuse but microscopic glow. The rumble of the trains and roaring claps of thunder always remained the most powerful sounds my ears could hear. No one knew I had a genetic abnormality which would significantly affect first my hearing and then my vision.

My mother told me that when I was old enough to romp and play I was always running off in search of fun things to do, which included crossing streets by myself. Distressed to tears, she would exclaim, "You're an impossible baby!" She related that I would grin impishly and mimic her stern words with, "potsy baby!" Because I couldn't hear my mother calling me from the distance, I received many spankings for being a "precocious but disobedient child." While I do not have memories of being with my father (my parents were separated when I was two), I was told he played the piano well. He would sit me on his lap in front of the Baby Grand keyboard, and try to nurture a talent that ran in the family. My mother soon realized, however, that music would not be a significant part of my life.

I vaguely remember my first and only piano recital. I was a ten-year-old, stricken with severe stage fright. Although I remember being shamefully embarrassed, I recall nothing of the aftermath. Neither Mother nor I had an inkling my first public appearance would "abort."

Mother had coached me on the proper way to approach and sit at the piano and now, as I had during rehearsal the day before, I sat straight, curved my slender fingers over the keys, and then it happened. Gracefully poised, my hands froze in midair! I must have looked ridiculous, and since I have always blushed easily, the color must have rushed crimson to my face. I was flustered and did not know what to do. Suddenly, I heard the audience clapping and felt Mother's firm hand on my arm, tugging me to get up and bow as though I had already rendered my little piece of music.

My biggest contribution to my mother was as a twelve-year-old "musician" when I kept day care youngsters entertained until their parents picked them up in late afternoon. Mother and grandmother ran a "nursery school" for a short time before our move to Florida in 1944. I was in the sixth grade. Every day after school I sat at the used upright that stood in a far corner of the children's playroom and banged to my heart's content. I played nursery rhymes to which my small charges recited in chorus (and off key) to my faltering rhythm. Most of the children were very young and could not pronounce my name, so they called me "Dossie." Cook Helen thought it was cute and started calling me by this nickname, and it wasn't long before Mother and my grandmother followed suit. "Dossie" was a pet name of endearment for me from then on. Mother only referred to my given name when she was either angry with me or wanting to be authoritative.

My countless visits to ear doctors were terrifying and painful. According to my mother, I screamed when air was blown into my ears, until she no longer could stand my anguish. Although time obliterated the pain of those visits to the doctor, I recall that I pled to "go potty," fervently hoping that somehow I would be extricated and forgotten in a toilet stall.

Finally, it became apparent to my mother that my treatments caused more suffering than the puzzling infection that plagued my left ear. After numerous appointments and consultations with several ear specialists, my mother refused to subject me to any more treatments.

I remember subway rides in New York City and hearing my mother's voice over the incessant low whine as the train raced through the dark tunnels. On the street, vibrations of the overhead elevated trains afforded me the same luxury, even though the din of congested traffic was earsplitting. Drivers of all sorts of vehicles communicated their own language through a constant staccato of beeps and blares.

In grade school I also recall lowering my head and placing an ear to the oaken desktop. The vibration of my female teacher's soft high-pitched voice sounded lower in tone and more understandable. I continued this unusual practice throughout high school but, of course, my classmates thought only that I was bored.

I am not concious of being adversely affected by my hearing loss at such a young age. I suppose you cannot miss something you never had. Educational literature consistently states that children who have RP from a very early age do much better psychologically than those who develop the disability during the important years of trying to develop their identity. Having a hearing loss since birth and then finding out about RP much later at twenty-five has only one drawback that I can pinpoint. I was much more reserved. I was not the center of attention for several reasons. I missed critical communication in chit-chat groups during recess, which I circumvented by involving myself in games that required more action than dialogue. As a twelve-year-old I stood just under six feet tall and was very self-conscious around my peers, a number of them much shorter than I. I never raised my hand in class because I usually failed to hear well enough to participate in group discussion. Most of my socialization skills centered around adults, especially my doting grandparents. Thank goodness I possessed a resourceful mind and an imaginative spirit!

Sometimes I wonder if Mother would have raised me differently had she known and understood the implications of a future manifestation of RP. Would she still have yelled at me for running in the street? Would she have pampered or protected me? I think not, because Mother was a very no-nonsense person. It's hard to tell, however, what one might have done under different circumstances. In a way I am grateful that my hearing problem was attributed to something "normal" like childhood ear infections. However, it soon became evident that I did have sufficient hearing loss to adversely affect my personal speech and language development.

6

2.

YOUNG ADULTHOOD
Denial and Awareness

When I was a twelve-year-old, seventh-grader just starting junior high, the teachers determined that my speech was flawed, noticeably characterized by a dominant lisp, (imperfectly pronouncing "s" and "z" giving them a "th" sound.) I hated lipreading classes because I missed the attention of being a star basketball player. (I was the tallest seventh-grade girl and could easily shoot baskets.) Miss McClellan, my speechreading teacher, was every bit the stereotyped "old maid." Her features were lined and intertwined with wrinkles like a road map. They were always moving, except for the smile lines. Wide-eyed, her face was framed by a frizzy, thin mop of worn-out, reddish-orange hair, and her thin-lipped mouth was contorted into inconceivable shapes to form vowels and syllables. I was fascinated by her appearance and her spasmodic, guttural tones put me in a hypnotic-like state.

"Watch my mouth," she would say with emphasis. Her long nails matched the color of her pursed lips, and repeatedly she waggled the index finger directly in front of them. I do not remember others in the group, only Miss McClellan. God help us if we dared to look anywhere but at her lips. I hated it, but I learned well. Later, when I reached adulthood, I realized I had learned almost too well. I kept my eyes riveted on the lips.

The following year my mother uprooted me by moving to Florida. I was not yet adept at lipreading, and I had two

8

drawbacks to contend with from the start. First, as a Yankee used to more precise, clipped speech, I now had to learn how to comprehend a Southern drawl. The slow dragging of words and elongated ending sounds drove me crazy. Consequently, the impact this dialect made on my newly-learned ability to lipread was disastrous. Second, I had always been an "A" student, Here, though, in a small, laid back southern town in the Sunshine State, I had to adjust to different rules and another dialect. I was quickly relegated to the back of the room because of my height. I was devastated. I felt shunned and unwanted, and became despondent. I did not fit in with their way of life. I could not hear the teacher, and made inappropriate responses to schoolmates. I quickly learned about peer pressure but still could not cope, so I withdrew. Sitting in the back, I daydreamed, chewed gum, and doodled rather than finish assignments. I thought I was being ostracized and this was my way of rebelling against everyone. I could not sort out what was happening to my once orderly life.

My wise mother sent me back up north that fall to finish junior high school. I stayed with relatives, was assigned a seat close to the teacher's desk, and made lots of friends. My mother must have learned during my absence that I needed special attention. Upon my return in 1947, she enrolled me in a local Catholic academy where I received a superb education. I was graduated with honors in 1949 with a one-year scholarship award to attend a South Florida college for women.

The new classroom setting was much larger and a lot of my teacher's instructions and lectures were lost before they got to my ears. Shorthand class was impossible for me. I could not read lips and write at the same time. I struggled with determined fierceness, and my teacher tried to meet the problem halfway by standing close to me when she gave dictation assignments and tests. It was the first time in my life I was forced to accept defeat as a direct result of my hearing loss.

At about age twenty-one I considered wearing a hearing aid. I had an increasing difficulty keeping up with running conversation and was embarrassed by consistently making inapt statements. I made more "mistakes" and apologized them away with remarks such as, "Oh, I thought you said...," or, "I couldn't hear that part because of the noise behind me...," etc. My excuses became more sophisticated, but I wasn't fooling myself and did not like the facade. When I was younger, social conversation was more of a patter, a banter where "mistakes" were not thought of as inappropriate behavior. But now I was grown, about to face the world, and was expected to do my best. I wanted to "fix" the problem, but when I took one look at the size of the battery pack and learned where it was to be stored I didn't want any part of it. In the early 1950s a bulky body aid was the only hearing aid device on the market. Walking around with an advertised bulge in my chest, which anatomically could not conform to the normal curves of young womanhood, was not appealing. I was very distressed, but my priority at that age was to look good. I would get by, I told myself.

I soon found that my problems were just beginning. I filled out many job applications, but in spite of excellent qualifications and presenting myself well, I failed to find work as a typist. In fact, I didn't seem to be employable. Despondent, I discussed the situation with my mother. She asked what I was writing on the application form. All of the forms contained one question which asked if I had any physical defects. I had not thought that being truthful would be detrimental to finding proper employment. Mother was terse and precise, "Don't tell them. Just leave that area blank. It's none of their business, anyway."

I was stunned. She was right, of course, but suddenly I felt as though my hearing loss was the "bad" thing of the past which had come to claim its disrespect in writing. Here I was making my public debut, and I had to start by being deceptive. What did my hearing problem have to do with my ability to be a speed typist, anyway? But I took her advice. Besides, I learned long ago <u>never</u> to argue with my mother. On the next application I ignored the question and landed a job as a teletypesetter operator for a major newspaper.

Within the first year I advanced to being the highest salaried typist in the department. Satisfied that I had established myself as a valuable employee I felt I could confess "the lie." I waited until the timing was right. One day I sat at the machine finishing up a piece of copy and watched my boss as he and a friend chatted about 20 feet away. I lipread that they were discussing a golf game. I picked up my copy, wrapped it around the rolled up teletype tape and approached him slowly. The friend had just left the office and I said, "I didn't know you were a golfer."

Mr. Litton looked at me quizzically. "How'd you know that?"

"Oh, well, I'm a pretty good lipreader." I smiled demurely at him.

He blushed. "That's eavesdropping," he teased. "Where'd you learn to do that?"

He did not believe me at first. I tested him, "Let me ask you something. If you had known I had a hearing problem... a "defect"...would you have hired me?"

My boss looked down and, with apparent embarrassment, shuffled his feet before he replied. He lifted his head and gave me a contrite look.

"No, I have to be honest. I guess I wouldn't have."

"That's why I didn't tell you before." I smiled again. "Now do you want to fire me?"

"Of course not!" He picked up a handful of want ads

and said, "Here, get to work; we have a deadline!" (Case closed.)

I don't think attitudes have changed much, at this writing, twenty-seven years later.

The bombshell dropped on me four years later in May, 1957, when I was diagnosed as having retinitis pigmentosa. Now I was going to go blind! I told myself I would not be worth a plug nickel to anyone. Fortunately, I was able to escape to the waiting arms of a supportive husband-to-be. The following month Don and I were married, and we gained an instant family in partnership—four lively youngsters under five-years-old (three of his and one of mine by former marriages.) I did not have time to dwell on two Latin words which meant nothing to me. I knew I had a hearing problem. It was something tangible. I knew when I could not hear and had never fooled myself that I could not hear like others. But blindness? What was that? What I could not understand or justify through proof of reality in my daily life had to be a lie. I whisked away the bad thoughts and concentrated on juggling my attention between my busy career and a ready-made family and household.

12

3.

THE NEW WORLD OF SOUND
Adjustments and Trickery

A t thirty years of age subtle changes in the degree of natural light became increasingly annoying. Ever so slightly my eyesight was bending to adapt to an imperceptible loss of vision. Colors were not as bright, and nighttime and the dark were blacker than preceding years. Otherwise, the threat of blindness was a mere passing thought. My hearing loss, however, was becoming a very real impairment. I misunderstood what was said with growing frequency, and my husband and I often argued about what really was spoken as opposed to what I thought was said. I was absolutely miserable. I denied and protested for as long as I could. Nonetheless, I again seriously considered wearing hearing aids.

With the addition of two beautiful daughters born in 1958 and 1959, we had a "tribe" of six vivacious offspring ranging from two to ten years of age, I felt the need to show more responsibility to my family. How could I be authoritative to half a dozen lively children if I did not know what was happening to me? After much internal debate (and I really debate myself to tears on such personal issues), I reconciled that I had no choice if I wanted to be a responsible parent and a true partner to Don. It was time to end my career of "guessing games."

After an examination by an ear, nose and throat specialist, I was referred to a dealer who introduced me to hearing aids which could be attached to my eyeglass temples. The world I had been moving around in for more than three decades now burst into a profusion of sound. It was noise and song together. More than that, the profound utterances of life were like reading a good book and becoming involved with its characters. Now I was really <u>hearing</u>!

At first my voice seemed unnatural, as if it were not me, but someone speaking through me. My babies' squeals of laughter were shrill and reverberated on my eardrums, the way my eyes always flinched from a sudden jagged bolt of lightning. Oh my, I thought, shielding my ears with cupped hands. Do all children make so much noise? Absorption of street noises took time. I kept turning my aids up and down. Claps of thunder and revved-up vehicles all seemed ominously too close. I felt as though I was in imminent danger of being swallowed by noise.

Sound was deafening and for awhile made me quite nervous. I cringed and was jumpy for months, clutching my ears at all unfamiliar noises until the newness of full sound had subsided. I found myself thinking out loud as I reconciled myself to the clarity of how my voice now sounded.

I practiced different voice pitches and conscientiously listened to <u>how</u> words were spoken. I corrected the way I previously <u>had</u> pronounced some words, and practiced good diction. I noticed that my speech was slurred in pronouncing certain words. My "s" and "sh" sounds were the worst; "w's" and "r's" were uttered similarly, and noticeably incorrect. I went to a hearing and speech center for more training, which reminded me of my junior high lipreading classes.

I listened with fascination at everyday sonances—the drip of a leaky faucet, the tired whine of the refrigerator coming on periodically, the pitiful creak our front door made every time it was opened or closed (and which my husband insisted was purposely never fixed because he was able to keep track of who was coming or going.) Even now, with just the two of us, the front door sounds like the hinges need a good oiling. The twang of our screen door was a more raucous high-pitched sound that grated on my ears. Again, we always knew who was coming or leaving the premises.

From across the street I was able to hear my children playing. I captured their enjoyment at play like hearing the faint twinkling of bells from the distance. And the birds! They had their own language, from a glorious warbling I heard infrequently to the familiar twittering and caws of the more common species. I marveled at it all.

I was so overjoyed at "coming alive" that I wrote a testimonial in appreciation of the special services the hearing aid dispenser had performed for me. His attention was more than "making a sales pitch;" he gave me the gift of sound. My tribute to him titled, "To hear Again is to Live Again" is reprinted here:

I am thirty-years-old, and I have just begun to live. And I mean that in every sense of the word 'live.'

To be able to laugh with people, to know <u>what</u> *I am laughing about; to hear the chirping of birds; to hear my children laugh and cry, not just in the home, but down the street at play; to hear the ice cream truck coming from a block away; to have the very comfortable feeling that my husband no longer has to concentrate in helping me by being my ears, and last, but most important, to be able to do the things in life I've always wanted to do—this is living!*

Just a year ago, before I went to see Mr. Lowman I was nervous, tense, and constantly stayed away from all social functions—yes, even church, simply because I couldn't understand what was going on. Now, today, I am a successful sales representative, giving home parties around town, and being able to hear well has given me the opportunity to meet and enjoy the company of dozens of people every week.

To me, with a severe nerve loss which caused me to be almost deaf in the high pitches of sound, a hearing aid for both my ears seemed a marvel in itself, but I could not possibly have adjusted to the new world of sound without the patience and friendly guidance of Mr. Lowman, who not only is excellent in fitting all types of hearing aids, but is also genuinely interested in each and every patient's welfare and rehabilitation. He told me that it would take six months for me to adjust to my hearing aids. At first I didn't believe him; I just couldn't understand why I couldn't just put them on and walk out the door. I had many problems and questions during those six months and every time I consulted Mr. Lowman I realized a little more that he truly was interested. The point that I am trying to make is that adjustment is made so much more quickly and easily with a 'helping hand.'

I am really very happy to have the opportunity to let people know that they can be as fortunate as I. I don't mean just the adults either! Most important, the young people, even babies, can now be fitted successfully. When I was two-years-old a hearing aid was unheard of for me.

In this day and age, no one has to endure the mental and physical hardships of a hearing impairment.

Then came the reckoning!

Now that my ears were "fixed" with the purchase of two aids, I had to learn self-discipline in wearing them. My ears felt "closed up"—restricted. It was not easy and I began to wear them only when I had to hear. I was working at the time and had a part-time housekeeper. I remember her chastising me, "Mrs. Stiefel, if you don't put them aids in your ears you're never goin' to git used to 'em!" I took Rosa's warning as caring for my well-being, and with a weak smile and nod of the head, I meekly retrieved them. She was absolutely right, too.

My husband was not patient with me either. To him, wearing hearing aids was like taking a pill to cure the problem. I had faked comprehension for so long the habit was hard to break. We were still miscommunicating because I was still pretending.

"Turn the thing up if you can't hear me," he roared. Each time I became confused, felt the tears well up, and in suppressing them experienced a sickening tight little knot in my belly. It was Fear making its unannounced entry and tugging at me to play the game again. I thought I was going to be "normal," but turning up the hearing aids did not make things "all better." Amplification did not translate to understanding conversation!

Once again I reached for a way to compensate and to learn new tricks to keep up with running conversation. The disadvantage of amplification and, therefore, constantly being subjected to a higher noise level, was a negative in the restoration process. Getting used to irritating sounds was necessary to gain understanding of speech, and I kept telling myself that, indeed, I would get used to the raucous noise level. Not so. Turning up the aids was overkill. It wasn't that I could not hear; I just could not understand the words. They were like disjointed pieces which led to much misunderstanding. Hisses and explicit consonant sounds in the rapid, easy, rhythmic flow of language were as imperceptible to me as trying to recognize a picture puzzle which has lost too many of its critical linking pieces.

I followed people who walked away from me as they were talking. (I learned this trick from a friend who used to follow me around.) My husband remarked one day, "She sticks to you like a worried shadow." It became a ritual to turn the television set down and the lights up when company was in the house. I turned my aids up when background noise was low enough not to cause an added problem. I lent my better "working" ear next to people with whom I conversed.

Keeping up with a running conversation in a group is an acquired skill I call compensation trickery. It wasn't passed to me or recommended. I just picked it up as part of the "trade"—much like games that people resort to on stage in the public arena. For example:

Mock Surprise: "Oh, I don't believe it! Tell me that one again!" (Mouth agape and wide-eyed expression.) The person telling the story always repeated the punch line with more gusto to match my enthusiasm, which invariably assured me of understanding the humor the second time around.

But I wasn't so lucky with cover-up tactics in group settings. Much later in 1977 when I enrolled in college again and participated in a variety of discussion groups as a prerequisite for a Mental Health Associate degree, I had great difficulty in discerning what was being said. At that time I had worn hearing aids for fifteen years and should have mastered all of the "hear but don't understand" difficulties. However, too many distinctively different voices posed new problems, such as soft-voiced females, the mumblers and murmurers, and in general, unfamiliar accents. Texans have a notable twang, especially those from East Texas, quite unlike the southern drawl of Floridians and certainly nothing like the clipped speech of New Yorkers. In addition, a great number of the students were Hispanic, and I had an extremely hard time picking up their soft accent. Every day was a struggle. I contended with the "pieces" of communication and tried to sort them out. At this point I began to think of other ways to fill in the gaps. I became proficient at reading body language through one of these discussion groups called "Group Dynamics."

Hearing well requires listening intently. Have you noticed how much easier it is to "hear" when your eyes are closed? Although most of us lipread, focusing full attention on what is being said around you is not difficult if visual distractions do not divide your attention. By accident one day I discovered how unrelaxed I was when having to split my listening energy between both hearing and lipreading. To me, comprehending what has been said is like deciphering code. After understanding roughly thirty percent of what is spoken, I have to fill in the gaps. Usually after spending a few seconds guessing what I've just heard, then trying to internalize the <u>supposed</u> meaning, I realize that I missed much of the next sentence, sometimes just barely comprehending cue words.

What happens next is common, even for the average person, but I never realized <u>how</u> we take in and store information. As I try to analyze <u>and</u> internalize what I have just heard, I miss most of the <u>second</u> sentence; so rather than fall behind I focus on the third one. If it doesn't seem important, I don't try to fill in missing words. I simply attempt to keep on target for that all-important key statement. (I am aware this also involves what I really <u>want</u> to hear.) Because this makeshift system of mine has <u>obvious</u> flaws, I resort to "note-taping" wherever and whenever I can for accuracy and to obtain all the dialogue when I need background information for articles.

Amplification causes unsettling problems for the hearing aid user. Many people think that hearing aids bring about correctable hearing as glasses do for poor vision. Because my hearing loss is in the high frequency range, I am prone to turn the aids up so I can understand female voices better. In order to accomplish this, however, I also pick up too much ambient noise in lower frequencies resulting in an abusive noise level that produces unwanted stress. At this point, my brain's listening channels "go off the air."

Through trial and error I have found a happy medium in high-level noise exposure situations of social gatherings and crowds. I now lower my hearing aids to a more comfortable level and request soft-voiced females to speak up for me. I have found this approach much more acceptable. Besides being innovative about an aggravating problem, it has taught me to be assertive about my special needs.

After the ears become familiar with life's sounds, the turning up and down starts. The initiation is over. The sounds of life are old hat. Now I choose to hear what I want to hear. After all, I was an adept lipreader for years but had missed out on sounds. When my vision began to disturb my normal functional pattern I began to "listen" more carefully.

If a person has a hearing problem from birth, details become extremely important. I always did a lot of watching. I observed people, and I read continually. I feel I must have been an avid reader because my social skills were hampered by my inability to respond quickly. I sensed that my failure to be "alert" made me appear to be "slow" or different to others, and I felt unwanted as a friend. I found comfort as an only child by indentifying with others through books. I read under the bedcovers with a flashlight as a child; and as a young adult commuting 60 miles by bus to work, I read paperback books by a faint beam of light 20 inches overhead. After Don and I were married I devoured magazines and newspapers.

Then came the time when cataracts began to interfere with my daily performance of tasks. I was 34-years-old and pregnant with our third child. Objects were a little hazy; details escaped me. I was forced to slow down. I began to rely on sounds to subsidize visual acuteness. It became difficult to choose which of the two senses to use. Neither was in the best working order, and for the first time I felt I was losing control over both my life and the children entrusted to me while my husband was aboard ship. I was also becoming anxious about my personal safety.

In 1965 I was pregnant again and was told (erroneously) that my child could be born blind. I thought that my vision, worsening from bilateral cataracts, was being snuffed out by RP as had been predicted eight years earlier. About this time also, the quality of my hearing seemed to be diminishing. From this period of my life to the present, I became acutely aware of the compounded problems stemming from the deterioration of two major senses.

4.

A LESSON IN EMOTIONAL PAIN
A Night of Terror

O ne late summer evening in 1976 I was rudely awakened by a sense of urgency. Our bedroom door reverberated from violent pounding when everyone in the house should have been sleeping soundly. I heard an insistent murmur rising in crescendo and felt the mattress release my now wide-awake husband. Something was terribly wrong for him to respond so quickly. Without so much as a break in the rhythm of his spasmodic nasal snorts, Don has been known to sleep through howling winds and pelting rain of our turbulent gulf coast seasonal storms.

I heard the sound of a muffled voice from behind the closed door and my husband's agitated tone but unrecognizable response. The dialogue was tinged with panic. Which one of the children was it? I sat up and hastily fumbled for my cataract glasses and hearing aid while listening intently for clues. No lights were turned on. I pushed my aid's on-switch. Nothing happened. Why hasn't someone turned on the damned lights, I thought. I was fearful as I realized the hearing aid battery was dead. A replacement lay in my purse—out of my bedroom, down the long hall, through the den and into the kitchen...in the dark.

Footsteps and voices filled the hall. I was frightened. I could hear the noise but understand none of it. What should I do next? Intuition kept me from turning on a light, and I repressed the urge to call for someone to tell me what was happening. No one else had flipped on a light, and there

had to be a good reason. Slowly, with every ounce of con-
centration and drums beating inside my temples, I slid off
the bed side and stood up. As I approached the bedroom
doorway I extended my arms rigidly in front of me. Fear held
me in a vise-like grip. My body felt unnaturally inflexible as
I moved forward with wet palms that met coolness in the
pitch black hallway.

I heard snatches, "smashed," "slammed," "Donna's
car." My heart sunk. Something had happened to my daughter's Audi parked in front of the house. I had to hear more.
I placed the aid in my right ear and toyed with it some more.
There seemed to be a short in the circuitry. Sound was
erratic as the high-pitched squeal cut in and out. Ah, it's
not the battery. I experienced a twinge of relief as sound
flooded my ear. Immediately I felt more oriented and continued along the right wall toward the den with more
self-assurance. The dog was even quiet. I had completely
forgotten about Princess, our Manchester terrier. Our
almost-but-not-quite standard-sized pet resembled a minia-
ture Doberman Pinscher, and she guarded our home and
its boundaries with tenacity. No stranger dared to venture
near our home without her emitting vicious, throaty snarls.

Voices in crisp undertones let me know an intense discussion was taking place. A scraping sound to my left told
me someone was opening a window facing the street. A few
moments passed, and I knew the panic had subsided. Communication was now becoming more rhythmic.

"Where's Daddy?" I asked as I entered the den and
extended my hand toward the back of my husband's
recliner. The chair was comfortable, concrete, and familiar.
Its touch and my visual imagery of it quieted my disoriented
feelings of temporary physical dysfunction.

"Moving the car back," my youngest son shot back at
me. I heard what was said this time because Danny was yell-
ing into my face. I felt tense with distaste over him shouting
at me.

"What do you mean?...Where did it go?...What happened to it?" My questions ricocheted in the darkness. I faced a form I couldn't see but could smell and sensed movement by slight and sudden drafts of air in front of me. What I had been told still did not make sense to me. The pieces of words did not form an understandable picture in my mind. The lights were still off, and Princess had not made a sound. It occurred to me that she might have retreated to her favorite position under the dining table. After all, she received her cues from her master who evidently was in control of the situation. It was now obvious to me that the fate of my daughter's car was the object of everyone's distress. Click! My ear felt like a vacuum and I became dizzy as if I had lost my sense of balance. Vertigo. I shook my head and banged desperately on my aid. A rush of crackling static and a "Whoosh" silenced it completely. This must be a nightmare; it cannot be happening.

Anger and tears sprang at once. "Will someone please tell me what the hell is going on?" My voice sounded strange, not loud enough, almost as though my throat could not utter the words. I yelled, "What is the matter with Donna's car?" Another dull thud. It was the front door again. I felt spurts of coolness brushing me, then a caressing hand made its way around my left shoulder.

"It's all right," Donna said, patting my back reassuringly. "Someone hit my car from behind. We're leaving lights off so we can see outside in case the hit-and-run driver comes back." I remember someone said that the Audi was pushed by another car into the next driveway. My imagination went into high gear as I conjured my own picture of what had happened. I could see it having jumped our curb as the driver of another vehicle ploughed into it from behind. I imagined tread marks, huge tracking dents in our rain-soaked front lawn and a tangled vehicle now resting in our next-door neighbor's driveway. Incredulous, I thought, of my mind's vision.

"What did they do to your car?" I asked in a hoarse whisper. A pat on the hand in the darkness, a resounding muffled thump of the front door, and Donna was gone. I wrestled with the hearing aid again then jerked it out. Poor Donna. And where was Don? Did someone see the accident and go off in hot pursuit of the offender? What about the police? The questions rolled in my mind while I tried to resolve what my eyes and ears could not. My thoughts churned. The thud again.

"Don?" Recklessly, I turned and switched on a table lamp by his chair. I saw his outline and turned to confront him. "Did you call the police?"

"What good would that do?" he replied, apparently annoyed with my question.

"What do you mean, what good would it do?" I was becoming hysterical. I stood on the edge of this horrible scenario, denied active participation in it. I felt useless and inadequate. Despair was conquering me when I felt a slow, burning anger rise, and then the rage came. My normal channels of communication had been cut off, and I had been ignored as if nonexistent for the past twenty minutes. In an impulsive fit, I screamed at my husband, "If it was your car, you'd be tearing down the street after them!"

"Let Donna call the police. It's her car," he responded resolutely. He slumped heavily into his recliner. I stared blankly at him. None of this was real. The players on the stage were not responding appropriately. I was confused and disoriented, both physically and emotionally, and sat down. Shock weaved its cocoon, shutting out all but my jumbled thoughts. Someone has just killed a dream. Donna had planned to sell her car for nursing school tuition money. No one seemed to care. I started to cry, my sobs sounding mute on my ears, but tiny nerve endings felt the prodding of tears as they trickled downward. When was the last time I had cried this much?

I still held the crippled ear-piece as I made my way back to the bedroom. I sat on the edge of the bed and blew my nose, air popping through my nerve-deafened ears. I didn't want to think anymore. That was it; I was crying to block out any more thoughts. My eyes were swelling. Damn! That meant I would not be able to wear my contact lenses comfortably for the next two days. I wailed even more. Who cares? My anger flared again, a smoldering coal midst the grief. How dare he not go out there to try and track down that hit-and-run driver? If it had been me I would have been on the Citizen's Band radio—that quick! I blew my nose again. What was Donna going to do? Weariness tugged at me. Under normal circumstances I would have called the police and asked them to check the area. How many vehicles would be out at 1:15 a.m. with a bashed front end speckled with blue paint? Damn my inability to be on top of things at a time like this!

Calm gradually came over me as I recounted events of the past hour. I remembered my paranoia while sitting in the darkness, not seeing nor hearing. What a disaster. It was worse than what had happened to the car. I thought about what Don had said to me. I reflected on the number of times I had heard him tell Donna not to park in front of the house. There had to be a simple explanation for the way Don had reacted to me. It was not like him. Donna did not seem upset with her Dad. Why was I?

With some effort I got up and walked down the long hall to the master bedroom mirror to examine my reflection. What a sight I was, red-splotched face and tear-streaked cheeks. I was through with the crying. Enough. How I hate myself for doing something so stupid. I even tried to transfer my anger to a defenseless object, I mused, glancing at the pitiful hearing aid which had abandoned me.

This had never happened to me before. It wasn't fair. I didn't even know if what I thought happened actually did take place. I was tired. I did not want to think about how

28

unlike myself I had been. I felt as if I had violated my own dignity and intelligence. To think that one little flick of a switch could wreak all this havoc. "Unbelievable," I said to my reflection and sighed. This must never happen again. Why, I could lose my sanity over a benign two-inch piece of ear equipment that had cut off my world for thirty minutes. One thing was certain. I could and would handle myself better in the future. I splashed cold water on my face, took a deep breath, looked sternly at myself, and said out loud, "This lesson is going to trail close behind you wherever you go, so you'd better get with it!"

5.

BITS AND PIECES
Glimpses of the "Madness"

Just as a picture is said to be worth a thousand words, these pieces of lives from around the world epitomize tragedy and isolation. Their thoughts are graphic and make no mistake that their feelings are real to those who struggle with Usher syndrome.

Their pieces of locked time are vignettes of a soul's mourning for understanding and peace of mind. Each of the following bits of troubled times contains a strong message, a request for help, a search for identity. I hope you will "look" at these "tarnished" treasures and let them teach you how much needs to be accomplished toward helping tear down the barriers of their self-imprisonment.

I wouldn't want to lose my uniqueness—even if it includes RP and hearing problems.

I am a very frustrated individual because I have not been able to integrate internal satisfaction with my intellectual capacity.

Doctors could only tell me that my field was changing slowly, no prognosis and no label, no ingredients, no nothing.

I became very obstinate, very determined and very tough-minded with demand for perfection.

Before I got married I told my wife: "I have a severe

hearing problem, and I don't know what I'll be like 15-20 years from now." I never told her about the visual problem because that would be asking for rejection.

It is much worse to be deaf than it is to be blind...when you're deaf you're shut off...when you're blind, you have the use of your hearing to carry on communication. But when you've got both problems it's an entirely different story...It's a coping process that has to be constantly reviewed, continuously changed, and always updated.

I can't follow conversations in crowded restaurants and dark places...it's difficult to ascertain facial expressions and get proper cues, but I'm adept at maneuvering food. I just make sure I don't eat and converse at the same time!

Living with a hearing loss and RP has been a constant struggle since I was 10...I was emotionally unstable in my teens but I managed to suppress my feelings and strive to do things alone. But although I don't participate in social life much I know I must not become a recluse.

I don't mingle in groups much because I have problems communicating with the deaf. Because my vision is at five degrees, others have to stand twelve to twenty feet away from me so I can focus on their hands. This is an impossible situation because of people coming back and forth between us.

I really wish I could get married for it is not good for man to be alone, but I realize too well my limitation in competing with other males who can drive their own cars. Who wants to have a date with a stumbling bore? Maybe I'd do better to stick to friendships. Then I won't get hurt emotionally or physically.

Sometimes I panic coping with success. Somehow I feel that I am still alive and kicking!

It's a traumatic experience every time I eat in any dim-lighted cafeteria. It seems the light is more subdued now that I have had cataract surgery, and finding a table has caused considerable embarrassment.

My job is on the line, and it was suggested I go on pension...I don't know how I will survive with inflation rates...I'm under great tension because I want to continue working, and I think some workers are over-dramatizing my shortcomings. I feel like a lame-duck waiting for execution. I wish a mouthpiece like you were at my side in defense of my case.

The last one reflects the anguished feeling and desperate emotion that all humans share in their special time of need:

People with RP need someone, something to hold onto—like the woman in pain giving birth—they need someone close, right there, someone to cling to emotionally that day and everyday afterward until they can cope on their own.

32

6.

MOBILITY
One Step at a Time

I must confess that I have intense thoughts about mobility training and wonder if others have mutual feelings. I understand why many persons with RP resist the opportunity to learn how to get around better. The first line of defense is, "I don't need it...yet." Consider the rationale behind such denial. First, a large percentage of people with RP, including those with both hearing and vision problems, really do think they do not need orientation and mobility (O&M) training. The second consideration is that RP and moderate hearing loss, although a compounded disability, is invisible to the public eye. Acknowledgment is perceived as "not normal." The label of blindness and deafness is too overwhelming to share with "strangers."

I often argued for many years over the issue of safe and independent travel, versus depending on others or creating a perpetual hazard zone for myself wherever I went. I maintained it was "better" to forego independence and involve myself with the easy, familiar, "safe" territory. First, from personal experience let me warn you—there is no such thing as "safe ground." Second, self-imposed isolation weakens emotional stamina. You will develop a feeling of dread whenever you are faced with having to go anywhere on your own. Consequently, you are liable to become mentally and functionally reclusive. Doctor appointments, grocery shopping, or even going to visit someone in the hospital will seem too much effort on your part—hurdles to clear rather than simple activities of necessity or pleasure. Instead you will say, "Well, I just didn't have a way."

I slid very easily into this complacent pattern of choosing the familiar way out. My world was down-sized, and my home was my castle (actually more of a fortress). Within these boundaries I could maintain the same hectic pace I had been accustomed to for so long. I felt free and, I thought, secure and happy. But it was a "fool's paradise." When duties took me out of my comfortable environment, the twinges of panic and acute anxiety reduced me to limpness and drove me to palpitations at the same time. My mind did not want to admit what was happening, but my body was sending frightening signals. Then I realized that life was passing me by. My self-enforced confinement was doing me in.

One day not long ago I had a startling revelation. I was unable to recognize a part of town located not more than two miles from my house. Several areas had undergone architectural change due to economic growth and had transformed a whole section of landmarked suburb into totally unfamiliar territory. It was an abrupt awakening that frightened me! I knew some dramatic changes were required of my sedentary lifestyle. I had to venture out, even if it was to the remodeled stores of a shopping mall I once recognized and frequented. This was terrifying to me. How could I have ever let this happen? It was time to get out more often. It was also time for intensive mobility training.

Attempts to teach me mobility skills go back many years. In 1965, our family was in New Jersey where my husband was assigned to a naval air duty station. Cataracts clouded my vision, and the situation was assumed to be an immediate threat of blindness. The State of New Jersey sent a social worker to evaluate my needs. Efforts to teach me basic mobility skills failed, and the home teacher taught my husband sighted guide skills so he could assist me properly. However, she did help tremendously by showing me better ways to handle household chores and to feel my way through what I could not see easily. She was totally blind, in fact the first blind person I had ever encountered, and I was very nervous around her during the first few visits. But she was personable and turned out to be a godsend in teaching me how to fasten clear plastic liners onto Playtex nursing bottles. They were tricky to maneuver and had to be handled under sterile conditions. It was the first household task I learned to master without eyesight. That year I received a card from the agency which certified me as legally blind.

Soon after we came back to Corpus Christi in 1967, a rehabilitation teacher came to visit me. I wanted to take a correspondence course in poetry from The Hadley School for the Blind. The first thing he did was to thrust a white cane in my hand and tell me I should use it. I waved it away saying, "I don't need that thing."

In the early 1970s I agreed to learn how to better utilize my residual vision through scanning techniques. I also learned how to use the senses of hearing, touch, and smell to accommodate diminishing eyesight. (At this time no one had focused on my hearing problem. I did not mention it, and they did not notice it because I was still an excellent lipreader.) I received orientation training at a downtown church. It was huge, airy, and architecturally squared off—a historic landmark facing the Corpus Christi Bay. It had lovely, large windows that gave me a wonderful view of the whitecaps sparkling in the sun. I could see farther away now since undergoing cataract surgery, but was bumping into people and objects close by.

I think the State Commission for the Blind must have posted a warning in my "dossier," "DO NOT APPROACH THIS CLIENT WITH A LONG WHITE CANE," because I did not even see one during this training period. I have clear memories of what was taught to me, and I enjoyed all the little tricks of using senses and learning skills other than for eyesight and hearing. While I did not like the blindfold it was fun to try it on <u>inside</u> the church where no one was watching. I soon discovered how sensitive my fingertips were. I was shown how to use my hands and digits to locate where I was, should I be faced with having to find my way around in a dim hotel corridor or even in my own home without lights. I derived great satisfaction from learning an alternative method that allowed me to function consistently no matter what the lighting situation was. This was the beginning of loosening my feelings of restraint about the world of blindness.

I learned my sense of direction by the feel of air currents around me. Still blindfolded, I recognized for the first time that losing the use of vision during this time actually heightened the reception of sound. I was curious about sounds I thought I did not know, only to discover they were noises I had heard many times before in other settings. Apparently I had paid little attention to them. I enjoyed the lessons that employed a sense of touch. I was taught how to trail on the walls, doors, pieces of furniture, dining table, and how to retrieve items from the floor.

After the blindfold was removed I insisted on going back to scrutinize everything I had touched. I have an uncanny feeling that life is perceived differently when explored through the five senses independently. The mental image of my perception of touch was different from that of visualization. My description of what I had touched was much more imaginative when blindfolded than when I merely glanced at it. I used cursory and short descriptive statements to describe what was seen. For instance, when I touched a keyhole I described its shape, texture, what immediately surrounded it, as well as the distance it was from the doorknob. When I peered at it, the keyhole resembled nothing more to me than a hole in which I could put a key to lock or unlock a door. I learned something important during this lesson. Without vision or hearing, sensations of touch and smell play a valuable role by enhancing feelings and imagination, not just to gather orientation clues.

When I finished examining all the nooks and crannies of the building, my next most important lesson began outdoors—how to check out where the elusive one-step areas were. I am always in mortal fear of turning my left ankle (weakened from past experience) at steps or "curbettes." Multiple steps and stairwells leading upward are not a bother to me. At least they are clearly in view as I gaze straight ahead and let my eyes follow them downward to find the bottom step. However, the reverse is much different; I have to look downward. Outside glare usually scatters light on the demarcation of each step's forward edge, which creates an illusion of a smooth, flat surface. I can not even tell when I have reached the last step. Of course I use railings to guide me but the fact that the steps elude me is frustrating.

My instructor showed me how to observe what multiple steps are attached to at the edges: the side of a building, a bannister or even grass, any of which probably would be noticeably contrasted in color. Steps stand out so much more clearly when their outline is seen from a side angle instead of looking straight down and ahead of you. After two months of sharpening my senses, I felt more confident to travel about for a while. I had twelve degrees of peripheral vision at the time and with the help of hearing aids thought I was once again on top of the world, completely able to get around safely.

In 1978, I again needed additional mobility training, this time administered on a large university campus. I had just received my associate degree in mental health and wanted to work on a bachelor's degree in psychology. I felt very secure at this point. I knew who I was and where I was going with my life. I picked up the telephone and requested training in the use of white cane travel by day and a heavy-duty flashlight for scanning purposes at night. Seasonal allergies were giving my left ear trouble again, and after recurring inflammations, my ear specialist advised me to leave the aid out of that ear. I had worn two aids seventeen years. Now I had to deal with the problem of imbalance, since I experienced a gentle pulling of my body to the right. This unnerving bout with vertigo made me nauseated and lightheaded at times, especially when I moved too quickly. But I was determined to overcome this dysfunction. I told myself I would get used to wearing just one hearing aid again, and I did. Compensation is a marvelous tool all humans possess. I have learned how well it works and capitalize on it whenever I can.

My new O&M instructor was a short, wiry, congenial fellow named Jim, and I wondered how he could protect me if I were to fall. But he was a powerhouse in O&M training. Because Jim had a wonderful, non-assuming personality, and because there was a ten-inch difference in our height, we bantered back and forth in a Mutt and Jeff routine that lessened any tensions. Once we "hit the trail," though, he didn't give me an inch, and I didn't dare overstep my boundaries.

We tackled crossing intersections at night in a nearby business area and full mobility on the rambling university campus. Jim told me I was to incorporate the use of my residual vision and hearing, as well as other senses, to familiarize myself with the spacious grounds. I really intended to use my cane on campus. After I had finished my training, though, and I registered for classes in the fall of 1978, I bowed to the offer of a friend to drive me to school twice a week. Conveniently, we attended the same classes, so just as conveniently she was my sighted guide. At least I realized it was important to have the cane with me. It was better to have it and not need it, than to need it and not have it.

At this time my lifestyle changed again when I became a full-time human services volunteer. I worked until midnight many evenings and stayed busy in my "cubbyhole"—a bedroom converted into an office. I spent many hours reading and handling correspondence and clerical work. Days flew by and Don did more of the daily chores alone so I could keep up with the rapidly growing group which was to become TARP. In 1982 I attended my first convention as a speaker, and Don accompanied me. For some time I had not ventured out alone, so my white cane was relegated to the back corner of a bureau drawer. I did not need it.

In the early 1980s I had even less time to think about travel, let alone to use my cane when I did go out. I suppose the idea could be construed as a guilty ploy when I tried to "endorse" the use of a long white cane. I asked a local television station to do a public awareness spot to tie in with White Cane Day on October 15th. The interview took place at a corner parking lot adjacent to a large chain grocery store. While the cameraman filmed me walking with my cane from the vehicle to the sidewalk of the store's main entrance, I was nearly side-swiped by a careless motorist. It was a great video clip for the 5 p.m. newscast, but the incident terrified me so that I put away the cane for good. I vowed not to use it again until the public was more aware of persons who use either white canes or dog guides. (One month earlier a dog guide was run over and killed by a local driver.)

During the latter 1980s my peripheral vision was down to four degrees, and I had a lot of trouble getting around, especially in crowds and mingling in social circles. I still wore only one aid and, as a result, was frequently annoyed by sporadic dizziness. Reality of where all this would lead jolted me. I could no longer push the ugly facts aside. Intellectually and functionally I now could see a real threat to my safety. I experienced more accidents in my home where everything was in its place and well memorized. I had no explanations, only the painful reminders. I tripped over my own feet, ran into corners of furniture which caused me to lose my balance, and had more falls. I regularly bumped into door jambs and complained to anyone within earshot (sometimes to no one) that either I was gaining weight or the doorways were shrinking. Still the denial—injected with poisoned humor!

At the beginning of 1988 I had a new tormentor—myself. What was I going to do? I slipped into depression and felt sorry for myself. I rationalized my woes, sorting out the demons I felt were lined up like a firing squad ready to take me permanently. No! I could see the entrapment; I had to get out. Not with a "guide," either. Ruefully, I smiled weakly and told myself that I owed an apology to my rusty, folded-up cane.

One month before, as if by design, a supportive friend had sent me a "Marshmallow Tip" for the end of my cane. This would enable the "stick" to glide back and forth in front of me instead of the regulation left-right Tap! Tap! that made me cringe with disdain. Now I could quietly, and by continuous contact, identify everything and eliminate undo attention. Don, scrutinizing me from the "wings," and noticing that I apparently accepted the cane, announced that I was to attend the American Council of the Blind convention by myself. I felt I was being thrown out on my own, but I took the "resignation" as his personal challenge to me. In all honesty I really did not have legitimate grounds to protest. That trip in the summer of 1988 began another chapter in my continuing battle over whether or not to use a cane. I could no longer function without one and, with my hearing problems compounding the safety issues of independent travel, I was forced to stand back and take a long hard look at what I was up against.

By January of 1990 I was ready for the next step in rehabilitation training, turning myself in for what I hoped would be a "new (functional) model." I would regain self-esteem and functional competency. I went through the same routines. I still harbored the same feelings. This time there was a slight difference. I no longer felt intimidated by my cane, but I wish I had come to terms with my "stick" many years before.

After a three-week period of general evaluation at Criss Cole Rehabilitation Center in Austin, I started basic mobility training in a small neighborhood setting. It was not easy to remember how to get back to the original starting point and equally difficult to reverse a route. I caught myself glancing around rather than trying to memorize landmarks. I directed all my scanning energy to areas close to me—the "straight and narrow." But I failed to identify sufficient clues as I went, or to count the number of blocks and turns I had to make. The problem partially was that I had never had sufficient peripheral vision to sharpen these skills naturally. For instance, a good driver relies on memorization skills, familiarization, and an acute roving eye. (My "career" as a driver began and ended within four years. I had not driven a car since 1963—twenty-seven years ago!)

At this time I believe that blindfold training once more, for at least a preliminary time period, would have been helpful and would have served a dual purpose. My impression, from talks I have had with professionals, is that they focus on utilizing remaining vision. However, I personally believe, particularly among those of us with hearing and sight impairments, that the blindfold technique has a certain benefit. Functional hearing does seem to sharpen when all attention is forced on listening. Also, I would have learned how to pay better attention to what my cane was "telling" me. Even a slight contour in the sidewalk can upset balance. My cane does not seem to pick up driveway slants, but I am told that I just have not learned to pay attention to the way the cane moves back and forth.

At other times an unfamiliar noise distracts me from thinking about where I am going. It is as though my two weakened senses battle for attention, and I do not always choose correctly which one to heed. My mobility instructor at the rehab center kept saying, "Let the cane tell you what information it is picking up." It seems that the "competitiveness" of seeing and hearing confounds me, decreasing my ability to assess imperceptible cane-tip vibrations.

I have asked persons with normal vision and hearing how they do "information-gathering." They all agree that they have to scan, too, when they hear a noise, but their peripheral vision picks up its source instantaneously. I suspect that the two senses of sight and hearing working together give us the most important "tools" by which to manage our lives. They operate as a team in that they automatically "cover" for each other. If someone is absorbed in thought, though, someone might be oblivious to sight or sound, but a panoramic view of the surroundings would soon snap a person's reverie. I miss all of this highly-tuned combination of seeing and hearing well. I must selectively search for that which is important at the moment. In doing so, I often lose or miss other information which may also be meaningful.

So, all in all, I feel strongly that I would have been much better off if I had learned the many safety measures when I still had a wider range of peripheral vision. Good habits would have been formed. Preciseness and self-discipline would have added grace to my movements with a cane. I have many regrets about my stubborness and obstinacy and inwardly cringed at others I met at the center who said to me, as I so many times said to others, "I don't need a cane...yet."

After returning home in March, a local O&M instructor named Judy began training me in all the areas I frequent or to which I have a desire to go once-in-a-while. Although having to use my cane does not bother me, parading my mistakes in public still distresses me. My worst mobility mishaps occur away from home in crowded places. This creates a mixed bag of feelings (to cane or not to cane!). Although I move freely around my home and immediate neighborhood, I remain guarded, almost distrustful, about my ability to move about well and safely.

One day recently, Judy asked me to select a recreational place for the focus of a mobility lesson. I decided to pick a route to the YWCA because I was involved in a walking program and considered swimming as a healthful adjunct. The jaunt to the "Y" is under two miles and takes approximately twenty minutes to travel (by cane!). For the most part it is an unimpeded "track," so relax, come with me and learn what an average mobility lesson is all about.

I am ready for Judy when the doorbell rings slightly before 10 a.m. I step out onto the front porch and check to see which sunglasses to use. (I have approximately five pairs of various tints to accommodate different times of the day and the sun's intensity. I am wearing contact lenses because I have better control over my natural, rather brisk, and long walking stride. I do not like to use my cataract glasses when I am out since the clearly defined viewing center is very small. If I turn my eyes from side to side, my view seems clouded as though I were walking in a fog. When I look down at the sidewalk my vision is blurred, and the distortion causes a little dizziness.

I choose a medium amber pair of sunshields, even though my dark amber sunglasses are probably more comfortable. It is a partly cloudy day, and the mid-morning sun is intermittently piercing through the spaces of low-lined clouds slowly crossing the eastern sky. The darker shades will not allow me to see well in tree-shaded areas. (Always try, at least, to minimize the predictables!) I put keys in one pocket and contact wetting solution in the other. My purse? I have learned to lighten the traveling load, since using a cane makes juggling "stuff" very difficult. Thank God for the "fanny pack!"

I am wearing a good pair of walking shoes, have applied sun screener, and, oh yes, my sun visor. I go back into the house for it. Even though I have wrap-around sunshields, a visor gives me great backup protection when I need to remove my glasses temporarily. I used to find amusement in the fact that an elderly friend wore a sunshade cap all the time, even in her home. It protected her from the glare of her bright overhead lights. I could not understand the benefit then; I do now. In fact, I wear one now and then to help eliminate unwanted glare when I am working at my computer. (Some days my eyes seem more sensitive to light.)

Before stepping off the porch, I unfold my cane and tap it twice against the sidewalk to make sure it is secure, then proceed as if I were alone. Judy will trail about two yards behind me. Out on the "strip" I experience immediate dazzle from glare. After about ten minutes the sun does not appear to be as bright as before. (Pupils do not accommodate to light and dark as quickly as for those with normal vision.)

I am watching for cracks and uneven places in the sidewalk, and low-lying limbs. (There are plenty of both in the neighborhood, and I am giving my eyes a good workout as I scan from left to right and up, then down quickly.) Judy says to let my cane catch the cracks, but I find myself directing my attention elsewhere — on the scenery around and ahead of me, scouting for recognition and places which may cause problems in a few moments. While she chides me for not paying attention to what my cane-tip is picking up, she tells me to relax, listen for cues, and scan for clues. "It's okay to use what vision you have," she assures me.

May's brisk winds make a whistling and roaring sound through my hearing aids, which are turned up so I can hear Judy who is tailing me about ten feet. I see a car ahead but missed the whirring idle of one in a driveway, ready to back out into the street. Luckily he saw me. Darn it! My vision had picked up something far away that wasn't as important as what I should have seen or heard close by. I hear Judy's voice again. "Use your ears <u>and</u> your vision."

I am trying, but becoming irritated. "Can't teach an old dog new tricks," I mutter. Distracted momentarily, a tree branch brushes the top of my head.

Judy catches up with me and advises me that the original route contains too many overhead tree limb obstructions, and I agree. I smile because the incident has jogged my memory of another obstacle course I encountered two months earlier at the rehabilitation center. I was purposely put on a route that was similar to going through a jungle — just to assess, I was told, what I could see and what I would do. The neighborhood section was a natural hazard zone. The O&M people could not have done a better job if they had planned it that way. I will never forget it. I literally used my cane as a machete to get through fallen branches lining the curb of a residential section that contained no sidewalk area. In addition, tree limbs sprawled out over curbs and obstructed my view, so I had to thrash through undergrowth and shield my head from the overhead obstacles all at the same time. But it was so unbelievable that I had a hilarious time bumbling through it all. What a setup!

Back from my reverie, we are now approaching a suburban business area, about a quarter-of-a-mile from the "Y." I am watching for many driveways. Some of them feel differently and have a small slope to them, just enough to cause a turned ankle. (Oh, another painful reminder, but I cannot allow myself to be distracted now.) Judy is reminding me to focus on the immediate environment and what my cane is picking up. I grimace. (I feel like a naughty child.) I am supposed to look, hear, feel, sense—do it together. I do not know how to incorporate all senses to function as a highly sophisticated, sensing, identifying, and locating system. How am I ever going to get out of this rut?

Absorbed by my jumbled thoughts I have passed about two dozen driveways and three parking lot entrances while doing all this. I am finally coming down the home stretch toward the "Y" building. (I have been here before, but under different circumstances.) As I come closer to it I notice lots of cars in a row. Parking lot! I see a building to the left and slow down. I see a walkway. (Actually it took shape in my mind because I knew for a fact it was there; otherwise it would have taken me longer to find it.) The grass, not yet green because of an unusually harsh winter, blends in with the hard-surfaced walk area. It is wide enough but not anything like the familiar squares of chalk-white concrete. I take my cane and poke it in the direction where I judge the border is, between the hard and soft surfaces. Bingo! "Very good," the voice says behind me.

When I reach the front of the building I turn and trail along it with the tip of my cane to find the front door. Once inside the building I remove my sunglasses quickly. I am scanning the area around me, trying to fit together memory and fact. My eyes are not adjusted yet to the unnatural and dimmer light. Everything looks very mute and drab. As my eyes continue to search for something light enough for me to see, I'm thinking this building is the pits for me. I look over the foyer area in search of the information desk. (Come on, eyes, brighten up!) Judy reminds me in a comforting voice, "Take your time. The building is not architecturally squared off to begin with." It is frustrating to try to orient myself, in dim lighting conditions, to a collection of irregular-sized wall and floor areas and then attempt to memorize their layout. Without perpendicular lines as a guide, it is a major feat for me to make each section in my mind an orderly part of a whole.

I am confused. I cannot recognize where I am, but I am walking slowly and looking around quickly. Ah, I see someone...sitting...at a desk! I am quickening my pace now and walk around the desk toward the locker room. I hear voices as I approach the doorway, so I am shortening my cane. I see a group of senior citizens getting ready to attend "arthaerobics" class, bustling and shouting back and forth with one another. I smile and say hello to them. I wonder if I were in the middle of this group how I would avoid slugging or tripping one of them with my cane. That's one lively bunch!

I am moving past them, and Judy advises me to stay close to the wall by tapping it as I go. I wince inwardly again, but do as she says and tap my way into all the nooks and crannies—rows of toilet and shower stalls, trailing along mirrors (almost ran into someone then...oops, that's my reflection.) I am trailing along another wall, and I do not know what the long, narrow ledge is. (Large objects up close are often unrecognizable.) Guessing my puzzlement, Judy says it is a "grooming" counter. It looks like I have made a circle of the locker room.

The group sounds quieter. Judy is telling me that the lockers are on my left along the entire wall. I begin to feel the cold metal and see a number. I bend over to read it. It is difficult, but I make out a number encased in plastic—29. I move my hand and eyes along to the next number—32. (I don't understand this.) I am moving on to the next one and it is 35. Wait a minute!

"Judy, why are these numbers in skipped sequences?"

"There are two short lockers and one long one to each section," she explains. The "piece" I saw and felt was the first of two lockers in a vertical row. The next row had one long locker. Still not believing what I have just been told, I physically glide the palm of my hand over the entire two rows to complete the picture. (Got it!)

If I had been an onlooker I would have thought the scenario a strange one. I had smiled and made eye contact with several of the ladies when entering the locker room just minutes before. If I could see them what was my problem with the lockers?

O&M training is a demanding learning process, as well as emotionally draining. The cane is a Number one deterrent to many persons with RP and with Usher syndrome. No one deliberately wants to be put in a "no control" situation, even if it is an experiential one where mistakes and fumbles come with the trade. I believe a certain mystique exists, albeit a negative one, concerning a "person with a cane." The picture is part of an old, invalid script, but it is still observed and incorporated—by both user and bystander.

All of this sacrifice in the name of learning to be independent? Is it really worth it?

YES!

I've experienced both sides of the fence—isolation versus freedom. All of it is vivid. All the emotions are real. The problem is alive and well and not to be minimized. I have already mentioned briefly the year Don "kicked" me out to fly on my own to the annual convention of the American Council of the Blind. How I hated every minute of getting there. The trip home was a piece of cake, though, and the next annual event was the epitomy of total independence—functionally and emotionally. What a glorious feeling to experience freedom of movement.

And how did the walk to and from the health center turn out? When I got home two hours later my sense of dread had already been transformed into a sense of accomplishment.

"How'd your lesson go today?" inquired hubby.

"Not too bad. But I'm still learning."

7.

TELLING SECRETS
Revealing the "Madness"

My dealing with the ambiguities of both RP and hearing loss are now well into the fifth decade. The problems and difficulties never go away, never get easier, and never seem resolvable. Subtle deterioration presents a slightly different set of problems—literally—every time I turn around. This degeneration is like a beautiful piece of recorded music which slowly has become tinny and scratchy from being played over and over by a once sharp but now very worn-out phonograph needle. Or, with tongue in cheek, like a commodity, I have shown considerable "depreciation" of sight and hearing over the last twenty-five years. In 1971 cataract surgery brought me supreme joy, a sense of reprieval, with 20/20 vision once again. It became a rebirth in many ways. Never again would I take for granted the gift of sight.

With the passage of time, the aging process accelerated and another round of complications began to impede my critical reading area of the macula. By 1988, seventeen years later, obvious changes were being recorded by ophthalmologists. The left eye experienced a "crinkling of the retina," a distortion that made it minimally functional. At that time I only had seven-degree "windows" with which to view my environment, and my right eye was forced to do all of my reading and close detail work.

Not more than a year had passed when my right eye suffered an abrupt maculopathy, causing irreversible incapacity to read. Ironically, I could still see but no longer read by conventional means. At this writing, the peepholes are marred, distortion is heightened, and my sense of perception is disconcerting and often depressing. Faulty perception has created a new ball park in which I must learn how to "pitch" and how to "catch" all over again.

Everyone at one time or another will experience a "crazy" moment, an optical illusion, or misjudge or misinterpret what is observed, but these tricky little deviances from the norm have become a very real part of the "madness" of my everyday life. I am misinterpreting much more often what I perceive to be happening around me. Incongruity and deceptive perceptions give me a troubling sense of fear that perhaps my mind is beginning to warp.

Recently I experienced one such episode of incorrect perception. My husband and I attended graduation ceremonies held at a local junior college auditorium. When we entered, it was apparent that the ceiling lights had been dimmed for the occasion. We chose two seats close to the stage where the orchestra musicians were practicing the entrance march. I kept moving my eyes around to try to accustom myself to decreased light and to see if I could catch a glimpse of something that made sense. I sat quietly for about twenty minutes to let my eyes adapt, then looked to the right. I saw someone I thought was my husband catching my glance. He had what appeared to be a bored, yet impatient look on his face as if to say, "Wish they'd hurry up and start." Spontaneously, I responded by shrugging my shoulders, rolling my eyes, shaking my head, then giggling a little, turned away. When I looked to the right again, the scene had changed. Don was sitting directly next to me! The first thing I said to myself was, "Oh my God, he's wearing a maroon, not a white shirt." Timidly, I peeked around the back of his seat. The man I had mistaken for Don was sitting in the second seat from me. Somehow, in a flash of trying to reconcile the distance, I must have thought Don had moved one seat further away, since <u>no other person was sitting next to me</u>. Wrong! At that moment, Don had leaned forward to speak to someone sitting in the seat in front of him. I had not seen or heard him because his dark shirt blended in with the dimness of the room, and the music had muted his voice.

This incident was a real emotional jolt! How could I have made such an error? How could I not remember Don was wearing a maroon shirt? How could I assume I was smiling at Don and that he was next to me when it should have been obvious that the stranger was not that close to me? (Both men, however, had white hair and wore dark-rimmed glasses.) My heart was thumping, and my hands felt clammy. I must be careful. This will make me crazy!

Years ago when these episodes were infrequent, I thought they were funny enough to repeat them as anecdotes to others who also recognized the humor in them. There were times when I was caught talking to mannequins, poles, or empty chairs. Then there was a more serious discrepancy of perception. I had just entered the waiting room of an unfamiliar doctor's office where my eyes fell on a beautiful blue-eyed baby being held by an apparently doting grandfather. The little tot seemed to have her eyes fastened on me. I waved, making funny, impish faces, hoping to coax a smile from her, but she never moved a muscle. Suddenly it dawned on me that the child was part of a large wooden-framed oil portrait. Discovering my foolish mistake, I darted my eyes around the room to see if anyone had witnessed what would have been regarded as very strange and inappropriate behavior. I was alone.

The auditorium experience could have borne unwanted repercussions if I had displayed my usual playful mood as it appeared to me. I could have teased this stranger with a seductive remark like "What are you doing way over there?" At this point Don probably would have turned to ask who

I thought I was talking to. The innocent onlooker certainly would have thought my actions odd.

I am developing a wariness in observing my immediate surroundings, mindful of the alarming increase in the number of quirky perceptions I have had from day to day. One of the most recent "mistakes" took place during an O&M lesson with Karyl, my current instructor. It was late afternoon when shadows had faded, and the sun appeared to be balancing itself on the dusty purple horizon.

While I walked along a side street, I remarked to Karyl that the German Shepherd I had spotted in the middle of the street was going to get run over. I continued walking, conscious of stepping on countless small twigs directly in my path. They made crackling and snapping noises, and I was absorbed in listening to the sounds. Suddenly I heard a louder crunch coming from the middle of the street just behind me. The dog! I swung around just in time to notice a car go by and watch the shepherd's lumbering body move toward the curb in front of me.

"It's a wonder he didn't get hit," I remarked to Karyl.

"Did you see what happened?"

"No, but it sounded like the car went over a bunch of twigs and debris and it made enough racket to make the dog move," I surmised.

"No. What happened was that it was a police car, and the driver turned on the siren momentarily, just enough to scare the dog out of the middle of the street."

"It sure didn't sound like any siren I've ever heard ," I said, chastising myself out loud for making still <u>another</u> error in what had taken place.

"But I <u>saw</u> it, and I <u>heard</u> it at the same time, you didn't."

I thought about that. In fact, I stopped, turned around, and said to her, "I still can't believe how I am confused so much about what I think is happening with what actually is taking place. I never used to do this!" (Or maybe I have, and no one has ever corrected me. But then again, not many other people <u>know</u> about the debilitating effects of having a dual disability.)

Now I am less sure of myself than I ever thought possible, and I have to work diligently at maintaining a respectable semblance of self-confidence. I question my timing for responsive action in a social gathering and try to be alert to signs of paranoia. I make an extra effort to move around slowly, to study everything in sight, and make doubly sure that connecting pieces to a picture or figures in an important action scene are together as parts of a whole in a way that will clarify and validate what is being observed. In other words, instead of glancing at a scene, I analyze it. If the scenario doesn't "change" and makes sense, then it must be real.

I also take time to rationalize what this "madness" is all about and what its repercussions could be if I fail to get a handle on it. Perhaps the imagination fills in the gaps that faulty "seeing" leaves for the brain to sort out but fails to recognize. It may be that weakened light-sensing cells do not have enough energy to deliver coherent messages to the brain signifying what really is being seen. However, even a glimmer of light working through a malfunctioning "camera" still delivers a picture of <u>something</u>. I suspect that some sense of validity is attempted by the cognitive information-gathering system. I have caught myself shaking my head, denying what I have seen. On the other hand, I have been caught up with the imaginative illusion, bought into it, and then been shamefully embarrassed at the craziness the situation has caused.

Television commercials are another frustration. They appear without introduction and disappear before I have a chance to connect the "moving parts," and I certainly have more difficulty with unfamiliar advertisements. Sometimes I cannot make sense out of a picture and move my eyes away from the screen momentarily, listen for clues, then look again. This is a trick I learned long ago with optical illusion photographs in which a person is asked to find a hidden object in a scene on a picture postcard. Most of my friends fail to find a "secret object" because they concentrate too hard and long on one target. Looking away and back again or changing the viewing distance helps the eyes regroup and locate a different focal point.

Lately, I have employed this method to draw meaning from pictures, snapshots, paintings, and any stationary objects around me. I can no longer trust that what I am seeing is true reality. Losing the ability to make valid, perceptive judgments about what I have seen and/or heard makes me feel very vulnerable. Do I continue to interact normally and risk the emotional consequences of unsuitable behavior, or should I be more reticent, subdued, and avoid active socialization? To sum up my dilemma, the world at hand often appears "crazy" to me. Conversely, I may appear to be the ridiculous element to onlookers in an otherwise normal setting.

How awesome and frightening to watch yourself losing control of the real world and not have the skills to know how to keep up with or accommodate others who seem to be in the "fast lane." What happens to people who are "left behind?" I am appalled to discover that some persons with Usher syndrome reside in state institutions because "there isn't a better place." I am also disheartened to learn in 1990 that students with Usher syndrome are still being incorrectly labeled "learning disabled." Simply put, learning by conventional methods is hampered by the compounded problems of a dual disability. I shudder when I think what might have happened to me if I had not been sent to a private school by my mother and placed in the hands of an attentive and understanding teacher.

The message is clear. Those of us with a dual disability must become aware of our anomalies and teach others by sharing our experiences. Parents, also heavily burdened, must find the strength to reveal their own inadequacies to others. Together, all of us must make laypersons and professionals aware that the combination of our aberrant perceptions causes us to appear "chronically confused" or "mentally deficient." Again, our responsibility is to explain that the difficulties we have in assimilating information and understanding communication is due to the combination of our hearing and vision dysfunctions. If we do not become self-assertive advocates, our "madness" may be misinterpreted by everyone around us. The enigma of a dual disability of two major senses truly places us in double jeopardy.

8.

THE "TWILIGHT ZONE"
The Gray Area of Inconsistency

Each day the sun goes down, I die.

T he above quotation is taken from a letter recently received by a correspondent. It is a graphic and true reflection of feelings about having nightblindness.

Have you ever thought how a dual disability might affect your daily life? Which one, vision loss or hearing impairment, causes the most stress and anxiety? The professionals are quoted in literature as saying that the effects of having the combination of hearing and vision loss is worse than the sum of the two genetic disorders. It is referred to as a compounded disability. To use an analogy, for instance, compounded interest earns far more money over the years than simple interest. Usher syndrome causes far more problems over the years than if a person had only RP or only hearing loss. It does not get better. You will not reach a permanent plateau in adjustment. Just as money keeps accruing when left in a savings account, frustrations and difficulties of Usher syndrome will continue to mount over the years.

The first time I learned of this forewarning I thought about my own personal experiences for reference to a compounded situation. I wondered if the professionals had documented examples, but to my knowledge there is no clear-cut evidence, only subjective, anecdotal information, so I would like to share with you how my dual disability affects me.

It is not easy to separate the senses for any function or task which involves collecting information from my environment. I have lived with a dual disability for more than forty years now. I know I cannot gather all the important clues from my surroundings by utilizing just vision or relying solely on my hearing. In fact, most people incorporate any combination of the five senses that may be required for a given task. But, since I do not have all of my vision working for me, and I do not have all of my hearing to employ adequate information-gathering skills, this does create complications and inconsistencies in gaining reliable data. More and more often I feel unsure of what I am doing or how well or appropriately I am performing a job.

I believe my moderate hearing impairment causes more physical and mental distress than my inconsistent four-degree tunnel of sight. Fluctuating vision still allows me to tap into the fiber of life for clues, but when my hearing aids fail to work, or batteries suddenly wane, I am almost deaf to understandable speech and to sounds in the high frequency range. I can sum up my feelings in juxtaposition: I feel like the world is overpowering me when I am temporarily rendered functionally blind and that I have suddenly lost my identity—swallowed up. When I have lost amplification and cannot hear, I feel like I am the only one alive and that my space has ceased to exist. If I am near people when I cannot hear, I feel I have been abandoned. Perhaps the following incident which happened to me about ten years ago will serve to illustrate a typical compounded dilemma.

One morning while starting to prepare breakfast for myself, I realized my hearing aid battery had lost its power, and I did not have a replacement. Since the rest of the family was away from the house and not expected back soon, I decided to make the best of an awkward situation. Have you ever stopped to think about your own "house-sounds?"

They are very personal and give me accurate spatial clues. Usually I am not caught in such a predicament, but it does happen infrequently, and at these times I tend to avoid being around people. However, on this particular morning I was alone and hungry.

I felt very strange in a kitchen without familiar noises. The refrigerator was devoid of its erratic hum, and its door did not squeak its usual protest when I opened it. I could not hear my footsteps on the vinyl floor, but I heard an occasional car drive by and the incessant drone of an airplane overhead. The quietness of the house was oppressive.

The aroma of frying bacon was mouth watering, but I missed the degree of intensity the bacon strips were sizzling so that I would know when they had reached a preferred crispness. The frying pan was too dark to afford enough contrast. I could not tell when to turn over the strips. I thought it was strange that I was unaware I determine cooking time more by sound than by sight.

I could not hear the hissing sound of water coming to a boil. It was as if my kitchen work area was encased in an invisible bubble. Cooking a simple meal seemed so dull and uneventful. Bacon and water appeared to be going through the motions of change—not activity. How boring. Mindful of other tasks being performed simultaneously, I set myself a "spatial timer" for fear that next I would smell burnt bacon! I made a mental note to be aware of increased humidity being emitted from the rising steam. I would know when the water came to a rolling boil.

While all this was taking place, a glass of water tipped over on a nearby table. I never heard a tell-tale thump nor a splash, but I skidded in the puddle it had made on the floor. It was an unexpected shock and sensation to have an accident in silence! Quickly I searched with my hands to locate the source of the spill. Slowly I felt my way from the floor up the chair leg, onto the seat (there was the overturned plastic glass), then on up a dripping corner of the tablecloth, and finally to where the glass had overturned. By this time all of the table litter in its path was soaked.

It is eerie and frightening when your space loses its personality. It seems so empty, absent of life and energy. Moving around in an area without sufficient sight and hearing can become a precarious "touch and go" situation when things "disappear." A peephole of sight in a mute setting makes me feel empty and unstimulated. Random thoughts increase. Sometimes reality appears to be pulled from my grasp. Cognition decreases, and I feel that something will happen to my mind as well. This is what I call the "twilight zone."

Most of my exasperating experiences revolve around entering into the realm of approaching nightfall. I call it the "Cinderella syndrome" because if I don't get away from a social gathering which has started in daylight, and is now dimming quickly, I am in deep, functional trouble.

I have found myself in the Cinderella snare more times than I care to remember. At least most of my friends and some acquaintances have a fair idea why I see quite well during the day but virtually become blind when darkness falls. When I notice the sun starting to drop below the horizon I say, tongue in cheek, "Well, I'm going to have to leave now because if I don't I'll turn into a pumpkin." After the chuckles subside I explain in simple yet graphic terms, the seriousness of my dilemma.

"Use humor when it's bad," is taken wisely. These words reflect an unspoken cardinal rule for many people encountering frustration and moments of embarrassment. When you can't get out of a position that is certain to entrap you, a witty remark will respectably disengage you. Invariably, people will be amused (although most will not know why), but you will feel less "stupid" when everyone seems to be enjoying the joke.

Over the years I have noted a right way and an incorrect way to try to explain nightblindness to people. Perhaps the following example will prove helpful:

FACTUAL DESCRIPTION

"We all have two kinds of sensing cells for seeing. One group for daylight, and one group for nighttime and dim illumination. My low-light cells don't work very well because of a mis-coded gene. Also, I lip-read because I have a hearing loss. So, when I'm in the dark or in dim light it's difficult for me to either see or hear."

SEDUCTIVE EXPLANATION:

"I have a disease called retinitis pigmentosa and I am legally blind. I'm also hard of hearing, and I can't read lips when it's dark. So, I really don't like being out at night."

Both are true statements. However, the first one is explanatory as well as educational. The second one employs unfamiliar, non-descriptive words and sounds overwhelming.

I have found that giving factual, non-threatening information at the beginning often leads to a desire for more information. I am very cautious about using words which do not "show and tell" or "paint the picture."

Before I learned how to humorize a "bad" situation, my personality would shift gears at sundown. I would unobtrusively withdraw to a quiet corner until my escort (usually my husband), would come and rescue me.

I have a vivid recollection of one social event in particular. It was in the early 1980s, and a volunteer named Betty and I were invited to a political rally under the guise of "The Great Cookout." We arrived in early afternoon, and Betty and I made the rounds introducing ourselves to the guests. We walked from group to group, chatting and eating barbecued chicken and pinto beans. We were having a marvelous time. And then...here's the rest of the story as you visualize the scenario:

Outside, darkness began to permeate the large pavil-
ion, obliterating details of people, tables, chairs, palm trees
and the banquet table. Desperately, I tried to memorize the
layout. Country music and laughter now seemed annoying;
small groups of people were turning into blobs of dark
shadows. I fastened my eyes on an empty chair and walked
slowly to it, wondering where Betty was. I sat down and
folded my arms across my chest. My heart was pumping in
rhythm with the drummer, and a tight little knot rose in my
throat. I slumped in my seat. I had just turned into a "pumpkin." The line goes: "A pumpkin doesn't see; it doesn't hear;
it just sits."

I avoid most all social gatherings that take place outdoors unless I know for certain that options are open for me
to move to an indoor area of controlled lighting. Generally,
though, I pass up picnics and barbecues because it simply is not pleasurable recreation any longer. I do make an
exception for family picnics. There's always someone who
lends a hand to take me from A to B or who will bring a plate
of food to me.

Restaurants have a slightly different set of problems to
which a few rules of selectivity apply. When Don and I go
out for dinner we choose restaurants which have sufficient
or controlled lighting in the evening. Dinner time by natural
daylight and a window seat overlooking the Corpus Christi
Bay is most enjoyable to me. During the summer months
we have a wider selection of eating establishments to
choose from. However, what is pleasurable in July is dis-
couraging in November. A 7 o'clock dinner engagement
puts me in the "dark," so to speak, and I am faced with
another stressful situation. However, I learned to circumvent the problem of how to execute gracefulness and good
manners without depending entirely on vision.

During my recent two-month training at the rehab
center, I participated in an Eating Skills class. I was eager
to join this small group of six trainees because now I would

learn how to "have my cake and eat it, too" without drop-
ping it into my lap! I learned some very useful tips in
recognizing and handling food in dim light. The training
kitchen contained a dining area much like one would see
in a home. The "stage" was set to simulate the worst possible dining experience—dinner by candlelight.

All of the "dinner guests" were visually impaired or
blind, but I was the only hard-of-hearing person. The
scenario created a compounded problem for me since I
found it very difficult to listen to instructions over giggles
and a constant exchange of barbs. Our food, which was
unseen and purposely not identified was passed around in
a variety of dishes. I served myself a little from each dish.
I industriously "worked" at my plate while the others conversed light-heartedly. Have you ever maneuvered an
unwilling porkchop into a proper cutting position in the
dark, especially when it is slick with gravy and camouflaged
with neighboring food? It took me so long to eat what was
on my plate, and I expended so much energy in the art of
consuming it correctly that I was ready to wolf down another
meal. After completing the course I certainly knew what to
avoid ordering in a dimly lit eating establishment. Heading
up the unmanageables were all meat containing bones
(fried chicken as an acceptable "finger-licking" entree is
an exception), green peas, spaghetti, cherry tomatoes, and
rice. Jello is touted as being borderline tricky.

The "eating in the dark" routine is also like being in the
"twilight zone." Eating in public puts me at an awkward disadvantage, even among friends. My feeling of clumsiness
is compounded by the fact that I cannot read lips and I must
turn up the amplification of my hearing aid in order to hear
conversation. If I add this distress to all of the dinnerware
clatter and the jumble of ambient, mixed voices, I am functionally and emotionally worn to a frazzle.

Do I still go out to eat? Of course. But I am very selec-
tive. I determine when the "slow" time is for serving dinner.

I have "tagged" favorite seating areas (some tables are numbered and can be requested ahead of time), and I choose a table which has lighting directly overhead. Other considerations are contrast. For instance, one establishment my husband and I patronize uses white dishes served on a red or dark-colored tablecloth. Selecting a corner table minimizes ambient noise, and the quality of the occupants' conversation is better preserved. Also, a talk with the manager or a hostess may help obtain the service you need to make your dining out a pleasing event.

The difficulties I have mentioned in this chapter never cease. The examples were not shared to exert negativity on the reader. The experiences are real and must be dealt with accordingly. You, as an individual, must appraise each situation carefully to decide which places and functions to avoid. The bottom line is knowing, becoming aware of what creates your cutting edge, what wears you to limpness, what puts you in a dither so that you are unable to function properly. Giving up is not an answer. Learning how to circumvent problem areas constructively is the only sane way out of the "twilight zone."

9.

THE SEARCH FOR ANSWERS
A Testimonial

In the late 1970s little was known, even by medical professionals, about the link between RP and hearing loss. This was true even with the sizable number of patients seen by professionals in either of the two medical disciplines. More than ten years later little progress has been made toward teamwork between ophthalmologists and otorhinolaryngologists for properly diagnosing Usher syndrome Type II. The following testimonial is from a TARP member, one of my earliest associations with a person having the same genetic disorder as mine. Her experience reflects that of many others.

I was diagnosed as having RP at the age of twenty-seven. This answered many questions for me, and of course, raised ten times as many.

All during my childhood, my parents wondered why I was so clumsy. I can remember saying "...but I didn't see." Of course they were at a loss to understand.

My hearing problem was noticed right off, even before I started school. I began wearing glasses at the age of ten and a hearing aid at the age of twelve. The "ear" doctor's diagnosis of my hearing problem was "nerve deafness...nothing can help except a hearing aid."

I used to wonder how in the world people drove cars (especially at night). If everyone else "saw" things as I did, why wasn't the world one big car wreck?

When my twenty-year-old son was six months old I went to an optometrist to get new glasses. He was so concerned about the drastic change in my eyes from the previous year that he urged me to get an opinion from an ophthalmologist. I did. If I could remember who referred me I believe I'd go back to him and ask "what for?"

After a very extensive, thorough examination he shook his head and said "Honey, you have what is called nightblindness. There is nothing I can do for you."

After a divorce in early 1971 I began to focus more on taking care of myself. I knew <u>something</u> was wrong, but what? Being short of money, I kept putting off going to the doctor. In the summer of 1971 I met Tom, and we became engaged. I decided to see my ophthalmologist. I was so excited about my engagement that I wanted to tell the whole world. When I told the doctor he tried to be happy for my sake but asked, "Ellen, do you and your future husband plan to have children?" I thought this was an odd question coming from an eye doctor, but I told him that we did not. He then tried to explain my "condition" to me. All I can remember of that conversation is "Retinitis Pigmentosa...blindness...total in eight to ten years...hereditary ...best to not have more children...no help...no cure...blind...blind...blind."

No mention was made of the connection of RP to my hearing loss.

I left his office in a "blind" rage, angry with him for spoiling my happiness—NO! This could not, WOULD NOT, happen to ME! Not just as I was getting my life back together. I'd found a wonderful man to marry, but would he want to marry someone who was "going blind?" My heart told me "yes," but my brain and my logic said "Hell, No!"

I walked the 25 blocks to work, too impatient with the world to wait for a bus. I finished out the day, but by the time I got home I was numb.

After dinner was over and the children were in bed, my fiance came over. I told him what the doctor had said. I gave my engagement ring back to him, mumbling something terribly pious such as "don't want to put that kind of a burden on you." We were married a month later.

Seven years later I developed an ear infection and saw an ear specialist for the first time since the age of twelve. He was not a very tactful man. As a matter of fact, he was very abrupt and of few words. After examining me and reviewing my medical records I had given him, he said, "I guess you know you have Usher's syndrome."

I said, "No, what is that?"

His answer rang in my ears for days, "You'll go deaf when you go blind, probably in the near future," and just as abruptly he left the room.

More rage! Not my hearing, too! It's not fair! How could God do this to me? Wait, my parents did it, but no, they wouldn't do that. God did it, but He's supposed to be a God of Love and Mercy. Maybe I did something as a child that I wasn't supposed to do, and this was my punishment! But what terrible thing could I have done?

S O M E B O D Y   H E L P   M E ! !

Silence.

A couple of years later my sister mentioned the name of a lady in Corpus Christi, Texas and put me in touch with Dorothy Stiefel. From this walking ency-clopedia of information on RP/Usher's I learned what *little is known about this "thing." Shortly after Dorothy and I began corresponding, my family learned that my younger brother also has Usher's syndrome.*

He and his wife went to see a doctor specializing in genetic counseling to seek advice about whether or not they should have children and what their chances were of their children having the same "thing." This doctor was kind enough to send a letter to the immediate family members explaining what his conclusions were, and from this letter my family came to a better understanding of RP and what is now called the Usher syndrome.

It took several years before family members, parents, brothers, sister, grandparents, aunts, uncles and cousins could openly discuss this. Even today some avoid the subject. My Mom told me of the guilt feelings she and my Dad each suffered—not knowing which one had passed it on to two out of their four offspring.

10.

PASSING THE GENE—AND MORE
The Power of Family Dynamics

Loosely, and with tongue in cheek, those of us with RP refer to it as "The Thing." However, with it is carried a self-perpetuating burden of guilt and shame for parents, and blame and resentment for the person who has expressed the gene and now owns the onus of how to handle the fear of possibly passing it on. I have some considerations to share about this "baggage," especially since it relates to punishment—"sins of the fathers." The biblical chastisement is still alive and maintains its tenacious, moralizing hold on many world cultures. I feel sad for parents who spend a lifetime of remorse over a real or imagined wrongdoing and for the offspring who fail to deal with this age-old problem.

A turning point in my life was the day I talked to my mother by long distance telephone about twelve years ago. I had been married about twenty years, and I was updating Mother on my local junior college courses. I had also taken a special twelve-hour course entitled, "Genetics and You." Mother was immensely interested in how I managed to divide my energies between an active household of nine and a new career in volunteer work. When I started to explain what I had learned about <u>how</u> a genetic disorder is passed from one generation to the next she became very quiet. I had just finished telling her how much better I understood the laws of nature which govern genetic diseases and paraphrased the information by explaining that nature is like a giant roulette wheel and that my having RP was a chance happening.

At this point it had not been positively determined that I had Usher syndrome, so I simply told her the facts as I knew them. Mother was silent on the other end, and I could sense that she was hanging on every word almost to the extent of holding her breath. I told her slowly that <u>unknowingly</u> she and my father both carried one gene, the very same, identical gene for the recessive type, and I repeated this important information several times to clarify its meaning, "There was no way you and my father could have known this."

I had barely spoken the last couple of words when abruptly I heard a quivering voice through a burst of sobbing, "Oh my God, Dossie. And I thought you had blamed me all these years for having this problem with your eyes."

I was aghast! Until this moment I never knew that my mother had borne such a tormenting secret. My heart thumped for her pain, but all I could think of at the moment was to reassure her repeatedly and in several different ways that she could not possibly have prevented nature's course. I felt that I was playing a reverse role. Now I consoled my mother when she had never consoled me. Evidently her troubled thoughts had been shelved for many years. Her sobs did not subside, and I was slightly concerned.

"But Momma, that's foolish. Everything we have, including dimples, color of hair and eyes, big feet—all of it comes down through the genes. It's like eeny-meeny-miney-mo...to which one is this gene to go?" I forced a chuckle to try to let her know that all of this was not as grim as she might think. I did not, never did, and never would vent anger, resentment, or "dump the baggage" by inferring that my parents were responsible.

After I rang off I cried my own tears of relief. What if I had never had that conversation with my mother? What if she had taken this unworthy, senseless burden to the grave? How would I have dealt with that? About five years later I learned of the connection between my hearing problem and RP, and when I told my mother she digested the information much better. She was able to converse with me as she might have done with a friend about a serious health topic. Referring now to my many childhood ear infections, she said, "You know, I did my best. I took you to doctor after doctor, and when you were not getting better, for all the agony you were going through, I just couldn't justify it any longer."

"I understand, Mom. I really do. I would have done the same thing if it had been my own child." That was the last time we discussed "passing the gene."

At the time of my initial diagnosis I did not fully understand what "hereditary" meant. I knew only that it was "in the family." Much later I learned about genetic traits and that Usher syndrome is a recessive gene. I learned that "carrier" meant that each one of my children would inherit and "pass on" one gene for this disorder. It is important to remember that it takes a "double dose" (two identical genes, one from each parent) to manifest the symptoms. None of my children have been affected, and because the first symptom of Usher syndrome is hearing impairment, I know that none of my grandchildren are affected, either. I confess that I am grateful for my "ignorance" during most of my childbearing years. After obtaining a clear understanding of the laws of nature and receiving quality genetic counseling, I was spared much grief and confusion so many others continue to experience.

When life becomes unbearable man tends to blame tribulations on others and catastrophic events on God. It is easier to shift the "blame" or find a "whipping boy" than deal with it. But easy doesn't do it; it doesn't resolve the original problem. If bad feelings or "unspeakable" problems are never brought out into the open, the same maligned bugaboo—the secret—is passed on to the next generation, along with the no-fault gene.

I recently received a letter from a regular correspondent who said his friend cursed God for giving him the "disease." The mother was quoted as "beside herself" and begged for someone to help her son. I could almost feel the anguish myself. Unfortunately, the availability of quality genetic counseling still appears to be sadly lacking in many areas. Examples of similar multiple responses follow:

"The doctor told me that sterilization was the only way to prevent bringing a child with RP into the world." (The patient was married to a Catholic and after heeding her doctor's ill advice, her marriage was dissolved.)

"The doctor said don't even get married...then for sure I won't have children that will pass it on." (The patient did get married, however, but I was told that since adoption was not a compatible option, their marriage remained unproductive and empty. It was later determined that the patient did not have Usher syndrome.)

"If I have another baby and it has RP I'm afraid my husband will divorce me because he said that if any of the babies were defective he couldn't handle it and would leave."

"I've just never had any children because I didn't want to pass it on."

"I've already had two kids. I don't want to press my luck anymore."

Subjecting oneself to unwarranted feelings is self-defeating. It is not necessary to be unaware or unsure about the true facts of anyone's genetic trait. Everyone should be able to seek genetic counseling for qualified, correct information based on family pedigree or history. People must understand that child-bearing is a personal choice between two consenting partners who have the option to bring a child into the world with or without "risk" of "passing the gene."

Perhaps this is the basis for feelings of guilt or blame. I often remind myself that I once turned down a proposal of marriage because I had this "thing." I would not like to think where I would be today if I had denied myself the happiness of having a family. So the bottom line is <u>understanding</u> your personal needs and desires and following through with all the options and information you have gathered concerning them. When you make choices, you exert your right to the pursuit of happiness.

CLOSING WORDS

We must have the gift to identify ourselves with other persons, to relive their experience and to feel its conflicts as our own...in order that we shall feel in their lives what we know in our own: the human dilemma.
—Bronowski

Once upon a time it was not socially acceptable to become angry or to cry in public. And once upon a time persons who were "different" were supposed to hide their disabilities from the public eye. No more. A physical defect is only the shell of the true being, the physical cloak of all that someone can be.

Having a dual disability has also tagged me as not being "normal," being "handicapped," "impaired," "limited," "restricted," "deficient," etc. The list of negatives is endless but I have learned they are just labels of convenience for others to identify how we appear. It does not identify who we are, how we feel, nor what we want to do with our lives.

When people ask if I wish I were "normal," I honestly tell them "no," then I ask them what they think "normal" means. Rather than merely trying to survive, personal struggle and challenge has forced me to look within and to learn from others. I feel that I have become a realistic part of humanity. If I have helped someone by writing this book, I hope the message relayed is one of hope, self-understanding and peace.

ABOUT THE AUTHOR

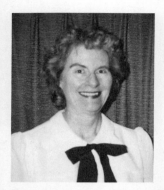

Dorothy Stiefel was born in 1931 in Mt. Vernon, New York. She was educated in New York and Florida schools and met and married a career Navy man in 1957.

In 1959 a Navy transfer moved her family to Corpus Christi, Texas where she divided her time between raising a family and continuing her career as a teletypesetter for a local newspaper. She also re-kindled her poetry writing. When her husband retired in 1967, the family decided to make Corpus Christi their permanent home.

In 1975 she organized a group for people with retinitis pigmentosa and a year later created the publication RP Messenger. Over the years the author has gained considerable exposure to the world of persons experiencing both RP and hearing loss and the issues confronting them. Although her human services work is a priority, she continues to travel and lecture when time permits.

After much urging from correspondents and friends, the author self-published two booklets in 1982 and 1986 as part of an ongoing series of publications dealing with personal experience and survival techniques. She states that this work and first book is a "culmination of a major chapter in my life."

Dorothy Stiefel has seven grown children and sixteen grandchildren and will be the first to tell you it is possible to be both a homemaker and a successful businesswoman in spite of insurmountable odds.

Other titles in the Business of Living series and available languages on 2-track audiocassette:

Dealing with the Threat of Loss, 1982 (Print)
ISBN 1-879518-00-7

Dealing with the Threat of Loss, 1983 (Tape)
ISBN 1-879518-01-5 (English)
ISBN 1-879518-02-3 (Spanish)
ISBN 1-879518-03-1 (French)

Stress and Well-Being, 1986 (Print)
ISBN 1-879518-04-x

Stress and Well-Being, 1986 (Tape)
ISBN 1-879518-05-8

The "Madness" of Usher's 1991 (Tape)
ISBN 1-879518-07-4

Type Specifications:
Helios Bold Caps and Lower Case for the text
Heads and subheads are Helios Bold Italic Caps
Typeset on a Compugraphic 8400 Phototypesetter

Printed by:
Grunwald Printing Co., Corpus Christi, Texas